DEFYING AGE,ANTI-AGING AND HEALTHY LIVING.

Staying healthier and younger for longer-Naturally

BY

KARO OLORI

entity with respect to any loss or damage caused or alleged to be caused directly or indirectly by this book.

It is strongly advised to consult a qualified health care specialist before making any amendments to one's diet or using the advice given in this book. This book does not replace or substitute professional medical advice.

IMPORTANT: Before commencing any major dietary or exercise routine changes or taking herbal remedies, consult your healthcare practitioner. Some herbs or foods might interfere with medication. If you are on any medication or a health condition, speak to your doctor before using any food, herb or activity suggested in this book.

Contents

INTRODUCTION

Technological advancements are slowly making it easier for humans to live longer. It is no doubt that we are now living longer than our predecessors. A few years back, it was not possible to live this long. Currently, approximately twenty percent of the world population is over 65 years of age. With this number set to multiply in the next coming years, most of us have a greater chance of living longer. This indeed is a great time to be alive. Or is it not?

We have succeeded in significantly increasing our life expectancy rate. Taking a deeper look at the older generation however, makes one wonder, if indeed this has been a good development. Yes, we have a number of elderly people now and more soon to join them. What purpose do these elderly citizens serve? Do they enjoy their lives? Are they comfortable? Do they continue being active contributors to society and the economy at large? The current picture is more gloomy than rosy.

Visiting a health care centre, one is quick to notice who the largest consumers of health care are – the elderly. As we get older, the risk of developing illnesses and diseases increases. A large number of degenerative conditions and disabilities are common in old age. The deteriorating health, the weak and feeble bodies and the burden these individuals end up being to society and to their family members makes aging such an undesirable experience. The deteriorating mental state adds to this discomfort. Most elderly people hardly enjoy their old years.

The medical world and scientists all over continue searching for anti-aging remedies. In their quest for solving this one mystery that has eluded human kind for centuries, they have unveiled a number of possible causes and contributors to aging. Indeed, there are some causes that we might not have a solution for. However, most of the contributors to aging can be controlled or at least altered and their harmful effects reduced.

Currently, a number of anti-aging remedies target only aging signs which people can see with their eyes. Given that aging affects a number of internal systems before the signs of aging are visible, these remedies are merely surface cures. Though they may improve the cosmetic appearance from without, they do not tackle the havoc looming within. In order to effectively reverse the effects of aging, an integrated approach, which addresses concerns from different body systems, is warranted.

There is no doubt that healthy habits and practices trump conventional treatments in many ways. There has never been a greater call to go back to nature for remedies and cures. Scientists all over the world agree that our planet and its natural resources hold the greatest secrets to wellbeing. The elixir of life, the elixir of youth, lies hidden deeply within the centre of natural plants and products. All we need to do is discover it.

In this book, we explore aging and how the effects of aging can be naturally tackled. It is the hope of this book to help each reader learn to alter their lifestyles in a way that will not only increase their chances of living longer but will ensure they continue leading healthy lives for longer. Starting with a brief outlook on aging, this book gives practical tips anyone can use to reduce the effects of cellular decline and unhealthy aging.

CHAPTER 1

DEFINING AGING

As we approach 40, the sad reality finally hits us -we are growing old! The skin stops being as plumb as it used to be. Streaks of grey start popping up. We console ourselves and name it wisdom. The so called wisdom slowly turns to ills and ails. Activity levels drop and simple tasks like standing up from a chair become a taxing exercise. As old age related diseases creep in, we discover that the painful end is upon us. What is really happening to a once youthful and active body?

Aging is a complex mix of biological processes which affect organs and systems, leading to various physiological, structural and functional body changes. These changes take place firstly at cellular level. The invisible effects are then translated to tissue, organs and systems and then become apparent on the outside. Appearance changes, muscle mass is reduced, bone density decreases, the metabolic rate starts dropping, memory function declines and a number of physiological functions including sight, hearing, kidney function, pulmonary function, immune function decline. The drop in immune function leaves the body susceptible to infections and diseases.

Many of us associate aging with the number of years a person has lived. Aging can be classified as chronological aging and physiological or biological aging. Chronological aging is associated with how old a person is. Some people can be chronologically old while their bodies look younger. Chronological age cannot be reversed. Physiological aging is not just a component of age as the number of years, it is a combination of age and declining physiological processes. There are cases where people can physiologically age faster than their chronological age.

Physiological aging results from some form of damage to cellular structures which prevents normal cell replenishment and repair. Factors that interfere with how cells are replenished or repaired or that contribute to the damage of micro-molecules would have a direct effect or influence on the aging process. While chronological aging cannot be reversed, physiological age can be controlled, reversed, slowed down or delayed by affecting or changing some of its contributing factors.

The reason we age has not been clearly understood. However, there are some theories and ideas that are widely accepted. One of the widely accepted ideas is that of DNA oxidation. The free radical theory proposes that aging results from oxidative damage to DNA which ultimately impairs cell function. There is evidence of premature aging in animals that have accelerated DNA damage.

Visible aging signs start showing after the age of 35. Aging however begins much earlier than that. Most human beings start aging around age 19. This is where most body processes start slowing down. Over time these changes culminate into the visible signs of aging.

Currently there are no known ways of reversing age. However the effects of physiological age can be reduced, minimized or completely eradicated by tackling a number of aging culprits. Our cells have an ability to renew and repair themselves. With age, this intricate ability is slowly lost. A way that can ensure the cell repair and renewal process is maintained for longer can be a solution to physiological aging.

Chapter Summary

Aging is a component of physiological as well as chronological aging. Physiological aging refers to the decline in bodily functions and chronological aging is the amount of years that have passed throughout a person's life. Aging starts earlier than we think and at age 19 the aging process already begins.

Many might argue that aging is a biologically programmed and eminent phenomenon. One consensus the scientific community holds is that, even if human beings are programmed to live for a certain amount of time, they do not have to be so plagued by disabilities associated with aging. Given that cells have an ability to self-repair, if we can keep them renewing for longer, we can in essence, slow down aging or delay its debilitating effects.

CHAPTER 2

AGING CULPRITS

Aging has a number of different causes. Among these are environmental factors, lifestyle, genetics, DNA damage as well as illnesses and diseases.

DNA Damage

Most of physiological decline and many illnesses can now be blamed on DNA damage. The role of DNA in illnesses has been broadly studied. Genes that control how we age do so by affecting how cells maintain and repair themselves. Normal cells follow a specific cycle of repair and replenishment. With DNA damage, this cell repair and replenishment cycle is affected.

Senescence, a condition where cells lose their power to divide, is thought to prevent damaged cells from proliferating. This condition is more prevalent in aging. Senescent cells tend to release chemicals or signals that cause other cells around them to also join them.

How DNA contributes to aging and the role of telomeres

Telomeres are looped structures found at the end of chromosomes. What has been observed is that as people age, the length of telomeres shorten thus increasing the likelihood of DNA damage. This might explain cellular damage in old age. Telomerase is an enzyme responsible for the production of telomeres. With age, telomerase production decreases. This contributes to the shortening of telomeres and the resultant chromosomal instability.

Environmental factors

The environment has a large influence on aging. The environment has been shown to have a big impact on modifying epigenetics and thus affecting aging. Inflammation and oxidative stress both which can be heightened by environmental factors are huge aging contributors.

UV radiation

The sun emits radiation which reaches the earth in the form of UV rays. These rays, though beneficial to most of life's processes are harmful, especially after prolonged exposure. The sun produces UVA, UVB and UVC rays. UVA and UVB rays are both damaging to the skin and contribute to premature aging which is also known as photo induced aging.

UV radiation affects the skin directly by causing photo aging. With skin being the major protective organ of the body, it is exposed to direct UV damage. The skin contains a natural chemical called melanin. Melanin is the skin's protective layer against the damaging effects of UV rays. When the body is repeatedly exposed to UV radiation than melanin can provide protection for, it can get damaged. Damage may include, fine lines and wrinkles, age spots, skin discolorations, dry rough and patchy skin and different types of skin cancer.

Pollution

There has been emerging interest on the effects of air pollution on skin and aging. Science has proven that many city dwellers where there are large amounts of air pollution, display higher signs of skin aging than their counterparts in less polluted areas. Polluted air is associated with a number of diseases including lung infections. Other toxins are introduced to our bodies through the food we eat. These greatly affect how quickly we age. With evidence of DNA damage as a result of free radicals and toxins overloading our systems, the role of pollution needs not to be ignored.

Heavy Metals

Heavy metals have been shown to have a direct effect on the aging process. The biggest culprits are iron, mercury and lead. These metals enhance inflammatory conditions and contribute towards oxidative stress and the resultant DNA damage. An over accumulation of these and other heavy metals to toxic levels has been linked to cellular aging as well as the development of some neurodegenerative conditions such as Parkinson's disease. Additionally, heavy metals interact with some proteins in the body causing them to malfunction. We get exposed to heavy metals through pollution, food, water, medicines and some industrial products and paints.

Oxidative Stress

Oxidative stress is an imbalance of oxidants and antioxidants. Common oxidants are reactive oxygen species such as super oxide anions, hydrogen peroxide and hydroxyl radicals. These can be produced inside or outside the body. When produced inside the body, oxidants cause cellular damage by damaging the mitochondria and other cellular structures. How a body responds to these free radicals has a major influence on aging.

Lifestyle

Lifestyle factors such as exercise, diet, caloric intake as well as certain supplements have been shown to affect aging. Lifestyle has a direct influence on how and when we age. Some compounds in the food we eat have a direct effect on aging. From contributing to certain age related diseases to contributing towards DNA damage, our diet plays a huge role in how we age.

The level of activity or inactivity also directly influences how quickly we age. As we age, many biological processes slow down. Energy levels drop and the resultant inactivity leads to a decrease in muscle mass. This further contributes towards decreased activity levels.Exercise has been shown to have a direct effect on aging. A sedentary lifestyle increases the risk of developing neurodegenerative disorders. Some lifestyle factors not mentioned above which have a direct effect on aging include:

- Poor diet
- Psychological factors
- Stress
- Intoxicating drugs and substances
- Drinking
- Smoking

Age related diseases

As people get older, they become prone to certain diseases such as cardiovascular diseases and neurodegenerative diseases. As a number of biological processes decline, the aging body becomes more prone to developing illnesses. With a decline in immune function, older people cannot fight off diseases and illnesses easily. These illnesses rapidly progress and in most cases become debilitating. Some diseases like diabetes, heart diseases and Alzheimer's are more prevalent in older people. Age related illnesses may lead to the development of further complications.

Inflammation

A common trait in individuals who live long is the ability to control inflammation. Some seem to have genes that protect them from inflammatory conditions. Inflammation is a huge risk factor in ageing. Conditions related to inflammation include cancers, cardiovascular diseases, Alzheimer's arthritis, autoimmune disorders, neurological disorders and pulmonary disorders.

Chapter conclusion

Aging is not something many look forward to. If you have ever had an elderly relative, you will realise the strain that aging places on them and on those around them. As mentioned earlier, the biggest challenge with aging is not chronological aging but it is the debilitating effects of physiological aging and the associated disabilities that arise as a result of health related concerns.

Many elderly people live with numerous pains as well as psychological problems. Among major concerns are neurodegenerative disorders with Alzheimer's being one of the dreaded age related conditions. Most age related conditions lead to a number of icapacitating disabilities, neurodegenerative disorders and ultimately death.

Aging is a component of many different factors especially those that lead to micro-cellular damage. As much as genes seem to have a larger role in aging, environmental factors, lifestyle and age related diseases and illnessess seem to be some contributing factors. An anti-aging solution which does not address these aging culprits may not provide a comprehensive and holistic solution.

CHAPTER 3

SURFACE CURES

As a number of people look for ways to delay the signs of aging, developments and inventions have made their way into the market. While most of these treatments promise cures to signs of aging, they target just the visible signs of aging. However, aging is more than skin deep.

Surface based oils and creams

Most cosmetic creams offer temporary relief and keep the skin looking younger and plumper. Moisture loss is more prominent as we get older. Good moisturisers can provide some benefit. A major challenge with manufactured beauty products is the number of toxins that might be present in these creams. Some creams are laden with heavy metals which are toxic and contribute to aging. What could be making you look younger on the surface might in fact be accelerating your aging from within. Natural based products without added chemicals /are beneficial.

Neurotoxin injections and fillers

These work by relaxing muscles in the face and treating aging lines. Fillers are chemicals injected under the skin to give the skin extra hydration, thus adding volume to fine lines and wrinkles and giving the skin a firmer and plumper appearance. These treatments fix the surface and never address underlying conditions. Undeniably, the temporary confidence boost is great.

Deep exfoliating treatments

Deep exfoliation treatments remove dead skin thus encouraging the growth of new cells. These treatments are widely popularised for removing dark spots and to even out complexion.Over and above the fact that these are just surface cures, there is mounting evidence that continuous trauma from deep exfoliating treatments can contribute towards aging.

Light based Treatments

Light treatments such as laser treatments are widely used for resurfacing, skin tightening and skin rejuvenation. These treatments are purported to renew the skin and remove skin imperfections. The safety of these treatments and their contribution towards aging and skin cancers is still being investigated.

Cosmetic Surgery

Plastic and cosmetic surgery is now common and well advanced. As with other cosmetic treatments, most cosmetic surgery treatments are merely surface cures. With decreased health and immune function prominent with old age, some of these cosmetic treatments expose the frail body to additional complications.

Chapter conclusion

A number of health systems are affected by aging. These systems include the circulatory system, the respiratory system, the nervous system, the excretory system, the muscular system, the skeletal system, the immune system and the integumentary system. Most anti-aging treatments tackle the skin which is only one of many different systems affected by aging. In seeking to treat appearances, some systems within the body might be sacrificed. Anti-aging treatments should therefore focus on tackling the entire system from the inside out with special focus on the cause.

CHAPTER 4

NATURAL DNA REPAIR

Repairing damaged DNA or protecting DNA from damage is one way to reverse or slow down aging. Our bodies know how to heal themselves. If cells are burdened with toxins, too much cellular damage or lack of the necessary building blocks and chemicals to repair, this process is compromised. If the body is supplied with the perfect conditions and resources to heal, DNA repair would be possible.

Food plays a massive role in DNA repair. By providing the body with adequate DNA repairing nutrients and antioxidants, DNA damage can be prevented, minimised or reversed. In order to effectively reduce DNA damage, the following steps need to be taken:

1. Eliminate toxins and reduce exposure.
2. Add nutrients and activities which aid detoxification.
3. Adding nutrients that help repair and protect DNA.

Reducing Toxins and free radical damage

Reducing exposure to toxins and toxic environments is the first step in preventing toxin overload. It is best to avoid food, water and environments with high levels of heavy metals. Filtering drinking water for heavy metals is recommended. When taking certain medication, it is important to find out if the medication does not contain heavy metals.

Most free radicals are produced in our bodies as by-products of the foods we ingest. In order to reduce exposure to free radicals, it is important to avoid foods high in oxidants such as processed foods, processed meats, oils, high glycaemic foods and alcohol. Replacing these foods with healthy alternatives will greatly reduce the oxidant burden in the body.

Foods which aid in detoxification

Fruits and vegetables have phytochemicals and flavonoids which assist our bodies produce more detoxification enzymes. Phytochemicals have been shown to modulate gene expression and DNA repair. Beneficial compounds in detoxification are found in onions, lettuce, green leafy vegetables, parsley, celery, citrus fruit, berries, cherries and plums. Other vegetables and fruits such as apples, red bell peppers, figs, pomegranates, beets, persimmons, spinach and prunes are also high in antioxidants. Spices such as turmeric, ginger, grape seed extract as well as rosemary also have high antioxidant properties. Citrus peels have been shown to facilitate DNA repair. Broccoli has also been shown to exhibit DNA repair properties. Apples have flavonoids which protect cells against damage and facilitate DNA repair. Strawberries contain ellagic acid which has both DNA protective and repair properties. Selenium, lycopene and zinc all have DNA repair and protective properties.

Chapter conclusion

A balanced diet rich in antioxidants, B vitamins, selenium, zinc and lycopene is helpful in repairing and minimising

DNA damage. In order to obtain the maximum benefits from most vegetables and fruits, it is better to eat them raw or lightly cooked.

CHAPTER 5

DIGESTIVE SUPPORT

The majority of nutrients supplied to the body come from the food we eat. The digestive system plays a huge role in absorption, digestion, dissolving and transporting these nutrients. In order for all the nutrients to be made available and beneficial to the various systems, it is important that the digestive system functions optimally.

The digestive system is made up of the mouth, oesophagus, the stomach, liver, small intestines, large intestines, the rectum and the anus. A number of factors can affect any part of the digestive system as we age. As much as digestive system disorders can occur at any age, their frequency increases with age. Digestive disorders include constipation, slower digestive processes, diverticulosis, ulcers, polyps, gastroesophageal reflux (GERD) among others.

Prevention is better than cure. A few steps one can take to insure a healthy gut include:

1. Eating healthy gut friendly food.

2. Incorporating fibre in the diet.

3. Increasing beneficial bacteria.

4. Avoiding foods that irritate the gut.

5. Drink enough water and fluids.

6. Treat symptoms as soon as they appear.

Gut healthy herbs

Foods, herbs and spices have been used for centuries to combat digestive system disorders. Some foods, herbs and spices that are commonly used are briefly discussed below.

- **Ginger:** Ginger has been widely used to alleviate nausea. Ginger contains among other compounds gingerol which is the main bioactive compound. Gingerol has anti-inflammatory and anti-oxidant properties. Ginger has been shown to relieve nausea and stomach upsets. Ginger is normally used as an ingredient in most dishes. It can also be used in tea, juices and smoothies. Ginger must be taken with care as large quantities might lead to stomach upsets.

- **Turmeric:** Turmeric is widely used to treat stomach ailments. Research shows it is effective in treating

Dyspepsia and ulcerative colitis. Its active component, curcumin is thought to aid digestion and enhances liver function. It is also reported to treat acid reflux and flatulence. Its benefits can be attributed to its anti-inflammatory properties and GI calming properties. As with other drugs, turmeric should be taken with care.

- **Milk thistle:** Milk thistle is commonly known as a liver tonic. It is commonly used for the treatment of hepatitis, liver cirrhosis and protects the liver from damage. Milk thistle has been shown to help regenerate the liver. Milk thistle has also been seen to be effective against a sluggish stomach. The main active ingredient of milk thistle is silymarine. There is extensive evidence that milk thistle is effective in regenerating the liver, protecting the liver from toxic damage and detoxing the liver and the gall bladder.

- **Slippery Elm:** Slippery elm contains mucilage, a gel like substance which coats the oesophagus and makes it perfect for treating and preventing digestive distress.

- **Pineapple extract:** Pineapple is purported to be a quick stomach remedy. Pineapples contain digestive enzymes which are highly beneficial in treating heartburn and indigestion.

- **Dietary fibre**: Dietary fibre fills you up with fewer calories and thus is beneficial for controlling caloric intake. Fibre has a low glycaemic load. Blood sugar does not rise too rapidly after ingesting a high fibre meal as compared to low fibre meals. It is recommended to take 25 to 35 grams of fibre a day.

- **Probiotics:** Probiotics are microorganisms which play a huge role in digesting cellulose, and keeping the stomach healthy by getting rid of unhealthy microorganisms. Fermented foods contain some strains of bacteria and can be very beneficial in improving the gut flora. Probiotics have been used in treating stomach upsets and constipation. Probiotics are also beneficial in the breaking down and absorption of some vitamins such as vitamin B 12. Probiotics are found in fermented foods such as yogurt, kefir, sauerkraut, tempeh, kombucha, pickles as well as traditional buttermilk.

Other steps one can take to ensure a healthy gut include:

- Increase glutamine and zinc levels. Glutamine is found in turkey, eggs, almonds, soybeans and has been shown to reduce leaky gut symptoms.
- Reduce the amount of red and processed meats.
- Never ignore symptoms. Always get symptoms checked out by a qualified health care professional.
- A number of foods, especially unhealthy foods tend to cause stomach upsets. Eliminating these offensive foods will provide relief.
- Avoid Stress. Stress has been shown to have adverse effects on the GI tract.
- Reduce the amount of additives in food. Additives such as salt, sugar and preservatives are not only bad for the gastro intestinal tract but they can contribute to other illnesses and diseases.
- Reduce the amount of trans fats. Like most additives, trans fats have been shown to increase

the risk of developing inflammatory bowel diseases.

- Avoid processed foods. Most of them contain way too much additives and trans fatty acids

- Avoid using artificial sweeteners. Studies show that some artificial sweeteners can cause bloating and an imbalance of intestinal gut bacteria.

- Mechanical digestion starts in the mouth. It is important to chew food and break it properly. When food is not chewed adequately, it can lead to poor nutrient absorption. Chewing food adequately mixes it thoroughly with saliva, which contains enzymes that break down starch and also aids food to pass smoothly down the alimentary canal. Indigestion and heartburn can also be greatly decreased by adequately chewing food.

CHAPTER 6

CARDIOVASCULAR SYSTEM SUPPORT

The cardiovascular system is one of the most important systems in the body. It is made up of the heart, the circulatory system and the circulating blood. The role of the circulatory system is to carry oxygen, nutrients and hormones to cells around the body and carry away waste products like carbon dioxide away from the cells. Other tissues and organs in the body rely on the nutrients and oxygen supply circulating in the body. The heart being a major organ of the cardiovascular system pumps blood around the body. If the circulation is not adequate, other systems in the body can be greatly affected.

A number of changes take place in the structure and function of the heart and blood vessels with age. The most notable changes are the thickening of the walls of the heart and the stiffening of the valves and blood vessels. The blood pumping mechanism becomes highly inefficient. The heart rate becomes slower and irregular heartbeats become common. There is normally an increase or a decrease in blood pressure as well. All of these factors increase susceptibility to a number of circulatory related illnesses which include hypertension, heart failure, anaemia and arteriosclerosis. A decrease in water content results in a decrease in blood volume.

A number of steps one can adopt in order to maintain a healthy cardiovascular system include:

1. Stress reduction
2. Exercise
3. Eliminating foods that are bad for the heart
4. Incorporating healthy heart foods and herbs.

Stress reduction

Stress has been shown to exert tremendous strain on the heart and blood vessels. When the body is under stress, stress hormones are produced. These stress hormones have adverse effects on the heart and blood vessels. Prolonged stress can lead to heart and blood vessel spasms, irregular heartbeats as well as an increase in blood pressure and heart rate. This may lead to stroke and heart attacks over time. Stress reduction techniques must be incorporated. These include:

- Exercise
- Eating a healthy diet
- Avoiding smoking and excessive drinking
- Practising mindfulness, taking time to meditate and pray and practising relaxation techniques
- Seeking the support from loved ones
- Practising gratitude

Exercise

Exercise strengthens the heart and facilitates the movement of oxygen and nutrient rich blood to other parts of the body. Adopting an exercise routine which includes cardiovascular exercises will greatly benefit the cardiovascular system.

Eliminating foods that are bad for the heart

Fast foods, sugary foods, processed foods, and fried foods rich in saturated fats are bad for the heart. Foods high in sodium are high contributors to cardiovascular diseases.

Avoiding these foods will do more good to your heart as you grow older.

Incorporating heart and circulation friendly foods and herbs

A number of fruits, vegetables, herbs and healthy oils are highly beneficial in maintaining a healthy cardiovascular system. Some of the beneficial plants and herbs are listed below.

- **Garlic** has been shown to lower cholesterol, lower blood pressure levels and improve the functioning of the cardiovascular system. Garlic contains allicin which is believed to keep arteries flexible. Garlic has also been shown to lower inflammation.
- **Hawthorn berry** in traditional Chinese medicine is used for digestive problems, heart failure, and high blood pressure. It is a source of polyphenols, which are potent antioxidants compounds found in plants. These help neutralize free radicals.
- **Flaxseed** helps control cholesterol levels and the build-up of plaque in the arteries. Flaxseed is rich in heart friendly omega 3 fatty acids.

- **Cayenne** enhances blood flow immediately upon ingestion.

- **Butcher's Broom** is widely used to reduce inflammation. This potent herb contains ruscogenin, which tones veins and enhance the flexibility of blood vessels.

- **Olive Leaf Extract** is abundant in antioxidants .

- **Bilberry leaves** contains anthocyanidin flavonoids which are potent antioxidantsand enhance circulation.

- Other heart friendly foods include berries, oats, legumes, beans, lentils, red wine, soy, colourful vegetables and dark chocolate.

Heart friendly vitamins and minerals

- **Omega 3** fatty acids are beneficial in supporting a healthy heart. Omega 3 rich sources include salmon, walnuts, sardines, chia seeds, mackerel and roasted soybeans.

- **Magnesium** naturally found in green leafy vegetables, whole grains and nuts has been proven to help maintain a healthy blood pressure. Foods rich in magnesium include spinach, avocado, nuts whole grains and some fish.

- **Coenzyme Q10**(CoQ10) is believed to assist blood vessels become flexible and keeps the lining of blood vessels healthy. CoQ10 can be found abundantly in meat sources, organ meats, fatty fish and some fruits and vegetables.

- **Vitamin D** has been shown to regulate blood pressure. Vitamin D is produced by our bodies when we are exposed to sunlight. Vitamin D can also be found in fatty fish, beef liver, egg yolk and some vitamin D fortified foods.

- **Vitamin K2** found mostly in green leafy vegetables has great benefits in reducing the risks of developing heart diseases by preventing calcium deposits in blood vessels.

- **L-arginine** is an amino acid that helps expand blood vessels and amplify blood flow. L-arginine is found abundantly in poultry, fish and dairy products.

- **Folic acid** helps lower risk of developing clots. Folic acid is abundantly found in vegetables which include broccoli, lentils, Brussels sprouts and asparagus.

- **Potassium** is known for regulating blood pressure levels. Potassium can be found abundantly in bananas and potatoes.

Conclusion

The cardiovascular system is an important part of our bodies. Maintaining a healthy cardiovascular system will ensure one is active for longer and will minimise the chances of developing debilitating heart and circulatory related conditions which are more common in old age. Regular exercise, avoiding stress and maintaining a diet high in nutrients which facilitate heart health is very beneficial.

CHAPTER 7

RESPIRATORY SYSTEM SUPPORT

The respiratory system controls how we take in and use oxygen in the body. The respiratory system consists of two major systems which are:

1. Cellular respiration which facilitates the movement and exchange of oxygen and carbon dioxide at cellular level. Oxygen is one of the key currencies in human cells. All major processes at cellular level need oxygen. In order for cells to function well, grow and heal they need oxygen. During the process of cellular respiration, carbon dioxide is released as a by-product. Carbon dioxide in high quantities is toxic to the cellular structure and thus it must be removed.

2. The pulmonary system facilitates the movement of oxygen and carbon dioxide in and out of the body or the exchange of gasses between man and the external environment. The lungs are specialised organs which facilitate this exchange. When we breathe in, our lungs take in oxygen which is

transported through the blood stream to various cells in the body. Lungs are made up of millions of air sacs which are surrounded by blood vessel where gas exchange takes place. Carbon dioxide circulating in the body is released through the lungs and breathed out.

As we get older, lung tissue begins to diminish. The number of air sacs (alveolar) as well as the capillaries around the lungs decreases. The lungs also gradually lose their elasticity and the muscles around the lungs get weaker. All these changes decrease overall lung function and oxygen levels. These respiratory changes make the elderly more susceptible to respiratory disorders which include pneumonia and bronchitis as well as the worsening of pre-existing conditions such as asthma. Airway collapse is quite common in the elderly. Reduced immune function also makes the elderly susceptible to a number of respiratory infections such as pneumonia and tuberculosis. Reduced cough reflex also makes it more difficult for phlegm to move out of the lungs. Pulmonary system changes have an effect on the entire body.

Maintaining healthy lungs will ensure there is an abundant supply of oxygen in the body thus maintaining the health of cellular structures for longer. Additionally, the lungs will continue being healthy and may fight diseases and infections easier.

There are a number of ways one can maintain a healthy functioning respiratory system.

- The first is to practise breathing adequately. Most people lose the function of some air sacs in their lungs because of poor breathing habits. Shallow breathing gradually reduces lung capacity. It is important to practise deep breathing.
- Exercise has wonderful benefits for the lungs and muscles surrounding the lungs. Additionally, exercising will ensure adequate oxygen transport to cells and facilitate the removal of carbon dioxide.
- Smoking is harmful to lungs and reduces lung capacity and increases chances of secondary lung infections. Second hand smoke is twice as dangerous. Even if one does not smoke,

continuously hanging around people who are smoking poses some threat.

- Avoiding polluted places will also greatly preserve the lungs and prevent the development of lung diseases.

- Use natural remedies to unblock airways and to keep airways healthy. Eucalyptus is commonly used for unblocking airways naturally.

- Get lung infections treated as soon as they appear. Lung infections can quickly become dangerous especially among the elderly. It is important to treat these infections before they spread or become life threatening.

Certain foods, minerals and vitamins are beneficial in maintaining healthy lungs. Some are briefly discussed below.

- **Rosemary** is a lung friendly herb and is abundant in vitamins and minerals which include vitamin C, magnesium, potassium, sodium, calcium and zinc.

- **Ginger** has been appearing in almost every section in this book. The benefits of ginger are numerous and some of its benefits stretch to the respiratory system. Ginger has been used over the centuries in improving lung health. Ginger can be boiled and infused in tea or added to smoothies or dishes when cooking.

- **Oregano** is a wonderful decongestant. Its properties can be attributed to carvacrol and rosmarinic. These two chemicals are good antihistamines and decongestants.
- **Teas** such as green tea are abundant in antioxidants. Infusing some of the herbs mentioned above in the teas may enhance their benefits.

Other foods that are beneficial in maintaining healthy lungs include leafy green vegetables, cherries, blueberries, olives, walnuts, beans and lentils.

Conclusion

Oxygen plays a major role in most processes in the body. Healthy lungs facilitate an adequate supply of oxygen while ensuring efficient removal of carbon dioxide. Respiratory conditions worsen with age. It is therefore

important to keep lungs healthy before any age based
complications creep in.

CHAPTER 8

INTEGUMENTARY SYSTEM SUPPORT

The integumentary system consists of the skin, hair, sweat glands, teeth and finger nails. The skin is the largest organ in the body. The skin protects the internal environment from external conditions. It protects the deeper tissues by providing a barrier to entering microorganisms and foreign bodies. It also acts as an insulator, thermal regulator and facilitates the production of vitamin D. Ultraviolet light stimulates production of inactive vitamin D in the skin. The liver and kidneys then activate vitamin D so that it is beneficial to the body. The skin protects the body from dangerous exposure such as heat and cold and prevents water loss. Melanin in the skin provides skin colour and protects underlying tissues from absorbing ultraviolet rays.

The skin, hair, nails and teeth being more visible to the outside world are what most people use to gauge aging. The skin easily displays signs of aging. The skin develops wrinkles, increased pigmentation and may sag. In some instances, the number of melanocytes may decrease. However the remaining cells may grow in size. Easy bruising is also very common among the elderly. The skin becomes very dry as a result of diminished sebaceous gland and sweat gland function. Another important concern to note is the reduced ability of the skins' function to regulate temperature as a result of the thinning of the subcutaneous fat layer.

Maintaining healthy skin needs a conscious effort and must be done before the signs of aging become visible. The steps below will assist in ensuring healthy skin from the inside out.

- **Increase water intake**. Our bodies are composed mostly of moisture. Drinking water provides cells with the moisture they need to stay plump and keeps the skin looking young. 8 glasses of filtered water a day will provide the body with the moisture it needs.
- **Avoid excessive sun exposure**. The sun is a huge contributor to skin damage. Avoiding excessive sun exposure and tanning beds will preserve the skin and possibly prevent the development of skin cancers.

- **Take care of damage early.** Whenever there are signs of damage on the skin hair and nails, treat the damage. Do not wait for damage to be excessive before you act.

- Include enough protein in your diet. Good protein sources include fish, poultry, eggs and soy.

- Avoid hash skin hair and nail treatments. These might you look beautiful now however they might have damaging long term effects.

- Avoid stress. Stress is harmful to many systems in the body including the skin. Stress is a common cause of many skin conditions. It can trigger inflammatory conditions such as eczema, rosacea, and psoriasis.

- Avoid inflammatory foods.

- Increase your intake of skin and hair friendly vitamins and minerals. Some include Vitamins A, C, D and E, Coenzyme Q10, Biotin, Manganese, Selenium, Copper and Omega 3 fatty acids.

- Include these hair and skin friendly foods in your diet:

  - Blueberries;

  - Fatty fish ;

  - Eggs ;

- Leafy vegetables;

- Oxidant rich colourful fruits and vegetables;

- Calcium rich foods such as milk and cheese and

- Healthy nuts, such as almonds

Skin care routines for younger looking skin

1. Keep your skin clean. Wash it with a natural pH balanced facial wash twice a day. Use your hands or a soft sponge instead of using a towel to wash. This will keep your skin smooth and wrinkle free.

2. Use a gentle exfoliator one to two times a week. Natural exfoliators free of chemicals such as oatmeal with yoghurt and rosewater will remove dead skin while nourishing your skin. Natural exfoliators will give you clearer looking skin without overly stripping the skin of its natural oils and protective barrier.

3. Natural fruits such as lemons are great at toning the skin, minimising pore size and ridding the skin of infection. Adding a few drops of lemon to water and rinsing your skin with it in the evenings will rid

the skin of harmful microorganisms while helping keep skin looking young and firm.

4. Use a rich natural moisturiser morning and evening. Keeping your skin well moisturised and hydrated will boost cell renewal and will keep your skin looking plump and younger for longer.

5. When washing or applying cream to your face, using upward strokes will keep the face looking younger for longer.

6. Avoid harsh soaps and face washes which contain sulphates. Sulphates strip the skin of its natural moisture dry the skin and quicken aging.

7. Practice face exercises. Face exercises will keep face muscles toned and will keep blood flow to the skin efficient.

A few tips and home remedies for great looking skin

❖ Honey is rich in antioxidants and has a number of amino acids, vitamins and minerals and enzymes. Honey is used in many skin care products because of its nourishing properties, anti-inflammatory qualities and its ability to facilitate cell renewal.

Both consuming honey and including it in your skin care routine will slow down the aging process.

❖ Turmeric has been widely used by Indian women to keep their skin looking younger, removing fine lines and wrinkles and to ward off infection. Applying it on the skin will give benefit. Including turmeric in the food will clear skin from the inside out.

❖ Oatmeal contains amazing exfoliating and cleansing properties and helps keep skin looking younger. Oatmeal contains healthy fat which make it a natural moisturiser and protects the skin from getting dry.

❖ Yoghurt is great for lightening dark sports and treating sun damage.

❖ In the past year, a lot of hype has been going on about coconut oil. Coconut oil keeps the skin looking smooth, plump and young. Coconut oil contains lauric acid which is an antimicrobial and potent antioxidant. Regular use of coconut oil will keep the skin looking younger for longer.

❖ Shear butter is a wonderful skin moisturiser which keeps skin looking young and plump. It is packed with amazing compound which make it reduce the appearance of fine lines and wrinkles and keeps skin looking and feeling youthful.

❖ Lemons have powerful antitoxin properties and help to remove dark spots and wrinkles. Using lemon juice directly on the skin will help lighten dark sports and will ease wrinkles.

The number of natural products is so abundant that this section warrants a book of its own. The book –"Skin Deep: Healthy Skin From The Inside Out" by Karo Olori contains more tips and recipes for younger looking youthful skin.

CHAPTER 9

NERVOUS SYSTEM SUPPORT AND CURES

The nervous system is one of the two major communication systems in the human body. The nervous system is a fast and quick acting system. The nervous system controls activities that we see such as smiling and walking, as well as activities we cannot clearly see such as feelings, emotions and memory.

The nervous system is made up of two parts which are the central nervous system and the peripheral nervous system. The central nervous system is made up of the brain and the spinal cord. The peripheral nervous system is composed of nerves connecting the brain or the spinal cord to other parts of the body.

Neurons are the basic cells of the nervous system. These generate electric impulses or signals which are transported from one cell to another. These signals in some cases facilitate the release of chemicals known as neurotransmitters which are communication chemicals.

Sensory receptors are located in many parts of the body. Our senses are part of this intricate system. Senses include somatic senses (feeling, pain, posture, temperature, pressure) as well as vision, hearing taste, and smell.

The brain and nervous tissue increases in mass during childhood and slowly starts decreasing during adulthood. After the age of 80 the decrease is quite rapid. Communication within the brain is affected with time. This is as a result of the wear and tear of the white matter region of the brain. The grey matter is also slowly worn out. Nerves and nerve ending deteriorate and most senses are affected. Way before symptoms appear, neurodegeneration would have begun and progressively declines with time. Symptoms only start appearing when too many neurons have been destroyed leading to what we know as neurodegenerative disorders such as Parkinson's disease and Alzheimer's.

There are a number of things that one can do to maintain a healthy nervous system. Some of these include:

❖ Sleeping well and stressing less

❖ Packing up on brain and nervous system friendly foods. These include:

- o Omega 3 rich fish and nuts. These protect the nerves from damage.
- o Dark green leafy vegetables.
- o Avocados are high in vitamins including vitamin k and folate which are well known for improving cognitive function.
- o Broccoli contains a compound called glucosinolates which has been shown to protect neurotransmitters from breaking down.
- o Eggs contain vitamin B and choline. Choline is beneficial for making neurotransmitters which aid in memory and brain cell communication.
- o Pumpkin seeds are high in magnesium, copper, iron zinc and powerful antioxidants that protect the body and brain from free radicals.

❖ Some herbs have been proven to be good for the nervous system. Some of these herbs include:

- o Milky Oat. Milky Oat is packed with vitamins and minerals. It calms and soothes the nervous system and has been shown to strengthen the nerves. It has a great calming effect on the entire body. Milky oat is beneficial for individuals under extreme stressful conditions.
- o Chamomile. Chamomile is widely known for its soothing and calming properties. Chamomile acts on both the central and the peripheral nervous system.
- o Passionflower. Passionflower has been proven to treat anxiety and acts as a natural sleeping remedy.
- o Holy Basil. Holy Basil is supportive to the nervous system by helping in stress reduction by supporting the adrenal glands.

CHAPTER 10

ENDOCRINE SYSTEM SUPPORT

The endocrine system is made up of glands (endocrine glands) which secrete hormones as well as hormone secreting cells on the heart, kidneys, the liver and the stomach lining.

Hormones are chemicals which serve as messengers in the body. They enter the bloodstream from their secretion points and are transported to their target cells. Target cells are cells that the particular hormone interacts with. Our bodies have a large number of endocrine glands. As much as some hormones control non-vital life processes like height and growth, some hormones control factors so important that the absence of these hormones would be life threatening.

Aging has a direct effect on endocrine tissue and endocrine activity. Hormone production is mostly affected and fewer hormones may be produced. Tissue becomes less responsive to the hormones that control them. Slower hormone metabolism and a slower rate of hormone production mostly characterized by a drop in oestrogen and prolactin in women and a drop in testosterone in males is common. This leads to the numerous hormone imbalance issues.

Hormones are made up of cholesterol. Consuming a diet high in healthy fats will ensure that the body has the basic building blocks for making hormones. Additionally a healthy diet rich in vitamins and minerals will provide the nutrients the body needs to keep the endocrine system functioning properly.

These 5 herbs have been shown to help balance hormones.

1. Maca is highly used by Peruvian people to regulate and balance hormones. It has been shown to stimulate the pituitary gland and the hypothalamus which all regulate other hormones.

2. Red Raspberry Leaf is a pleasant tasting herb which is known to strengthen the uterus in women. Rich in vitamins and minerals, red raspberry leaf is beneficial for hormonal balance in both males and females.

3. Chaste Tree Berry is widely used for regulating hormones, treating endometriosis, infertility and reduces the symptoms of menopause. Chaste tree berry also regulates the pituitary gland.

4. Milk Thistle has been discussed before for its liver regeneration properties. A healthy liver is essential for hormonal balance. Excess hormones are filtered out by the liver. In order to avoid excessive build-up of hormones in the blood stream a good functioning liver is essential.

CHAPTER 11

IMMUNE SYSTEM SUPPORT

The immune system and its cells protect the body and defend it against viruses, bacteria, fungi and certain parasites. It is also responsible for removing foreign substances and removing abnormal cells such as cancer cells. The immune system is made up of various cells which together perform these functions. These cells are found in the circulating blood, in lymph and in various tissues all over the body. The major cells of the immune system include white blood cells, plasma cells, macrophages as well as mast cells.

With age, immune function declines. This is partly as a result of the breaking down of the thymus, the gland where T cells mature. This results in a decline in T cell numbers. Other factors also contribute to a decline in B cells and other immune cells. The result is a weakened immune system. This leaves the aged body more susceptible to infectious diseases. Additionally ,the inflammatory response is heightened in aging.

Inflammatory conditions such as arthritis are more common.

Maintaining a healthy immune system will ensure the body can continue fighting off unwanted organisms later in life. Just like other systems, nutrition plays a huge role in ensuring a healthy and optimally functioning immune system. Nutrients beneficial for a healthy immune system are listed below:

- ❖ Good sources of protein will provide the body with essential amino acids to heal and recover. Good sources of protein include seafood, lean meat, poultry, eggs, beans, peas, soy products as well as seeds and nuts.

- ❖ Vitamin A is a great immune system regulator. It also has protective functions against infections. Vitamin A keeps the skin, the lining of the intestines and the lungs healthy. Foods that are high in vitamin A include sweet potatoes, carrots, broccoli, spinach, red bell peppers, apricots and eggs.

❖ Vitamin C is a good antioxidant and stimulates the formation of antibodies. Foods high in vitamin C include citrus fruits, red bell pepper, papaya, strawberries and tomatoes.

❖ Vitamin E is a wonderful antioxidant which can improve immune function. Vitamin E is abundant in sunflower seeds, almonds, and some nuts.

❖ Zinc modulates the immune system and facilitates wound healing. Zinc is found in animal products, seafood, whole grains, nuts and beans.

❖ Other nutrients such as vitamin Folate, Selenium and Iron can support the function of the immune system.

Immune boosting herbs include:

❖ Garlic

❖ Medicinal mushrooms

❖ Ginseng

❖ Astralagus

❖ Ginger

❖ Tumeric

- ❖ Echinacea
- ❖ Ginseng

CHAPTER 12

MUSCULO-SKELETAL SUPPORT

The musculo-skeletal system is responsible for posture and movement. The musculo-skeletal system is closely controlled by the nervous system.

With age, a decrease in muscle mass either as a result of reduction in activity and calorie intake has been observed. The bone marrow volume also has been shown to decrease as well as a reduction in mineral content and softening of the bones. The cartilage layer is not immune to the effects of aging. As stress is exerted on the cartilage layer it begins to deteriorate leading to degenerative cartilage diseases like osteoarthritis. As more of the cartilage extra-cellular matrix is degraded, underlying cartilage layers are also destroyed until bones grind against each other, a painful experience accompanied by inflammation.

One common age related condition is sarcopenia. Sarcopenia is a condition associated with muscle mass decline. At around age 30, muscles begin deteriorating.

This happens quicker in individuals who are less active. More active individuals may still lose some muscle but less gradually. At around age 75, muscle decline is more rapid. Low hormone levels have been linked to muscle decline.

Musculo-skeletal problems are very common with age. Some of the major ailments include back pain, arthritis, joint pain and osteoporosis. Some problems with musculo-skeletal conditions are a result of other underlying conditions while others result from pulled muscles and strained ligaments. In order to keep this system healthy and move easily till old age, a few simple steps can be taken.

- ❖ Yoga is well known for toning and strengthening bones, muscles and connective tissue. Yoga poses gently stretch muscles and make the body more flexible. Bone flexibility is also enhanced with yoga. Over and above the musculoskeletal benefits yoga is a great stress reliever.
- ❖ Exercise when done properly is highly beneficial for the skeleto-muscular system. Incorporating good exercise routines and stretches will greatly enhance and strengthen the skeleto-muscular

system. When exercising, it is important to take good care of muscles. Warming up before stretching will help prevent injuries.

- ❖ Incorporate food and herbs that strengthen the skeleto-muscular system. Herbs for a healthy skeleto-muscular system include:
  - o Turmeric
  - o Gotu kola
  - o Nettle leaf
  - o Seaweeds
  - o Burdock root
  - o Dandelion root.
- ❖ Vitamin D3 is important for bone health and may prevent osteoporosis.
- ❖ Magnesium is beneficial for a number of body processes including supporting bone health and muscle. Magnesium is found abundant in most dark pigmented vegetables
- ❖ Calcium is one of the most important minerals for bone health. Calcium is found in dairy products, and some green leafy vegetables.

CHAPTER 13

EXCRETORY SUPPORT

The excretory system is an important part of the body. Its major function is waste removal and fluid balance. The renal system is made up of a pair of kidneys, ureters, a bladder and the urethra. Kidneys play a crucial role in regulating water concentration, inorganic ions and the pH balance in the body. Kidneys do this by filtering out inorganic substances from the blood diluting and excreting these in urine. Another function that is not well known is the synthesis of glucose from amino acids during prolonged fasting periods.

Each person has a set of kidneys which are connected to a bladder through a set of urethras. The kidneys are made of a million nephrons where most filtration takes place. Blood flows through these structures in the kidneys and dissolved waste is filtered out and removed as urine.

The renal system is greatly affected by the aging processes. In some cases the filtering function of the kidneys is impaired as nephrons are gradually destroyed.

This causes an accumulation of waste products in the body. Bladder function is also affected by old age with the muscles of the bladder becoming loose. Incontinence is common with age.

There are a number of ways that can help keep the renal system healthy.

- Controlling blood sugar. Uncontrolled blood sugar has been shown to damage blood vessels.
- Control blood pressure. Like blood sugar, uncontrolled blood pressure has been shown to damage blood vessels.
- Healthy eating
- Drinking plenty of water
- Treating any pain or discomfort quickly
- Limiting the amounts of toxins and unnecessary medication
- Limiting exposure to environmental toxins
- Getting as much nutrients from food as possible and limiting supplements
- Reducing the amount of sodium in the diet

- If kidney function has been impaired, it is important to limit the amount of potassium and phosphorus and protein.

Some foods that are kidney friendly include:

- ❖ Cauliflower is a high in vitamin C, K and folate. It is also high in anti-inflammatory substances and is a good source of fibre.
- ❖ Blue berries are packed with kidney friendly antioxidants and are low in phosphorus and potassium.
- ❖ Red grapes are high in vitamin C and antioxidants and they have been shown to reduce inflammation. Egg whites are a great source of protein minus the high potassium present in egg yolk.
- ❖ Garlic not only adds flavour to food but it is high in vitamins B6, vitamin C and manganese. Garlic has great anti-inflammatory qualities which make it beneficial in kidney health.
- ❖ Cabbage is loaded with a number of kidney friendly vitamins like vitamin K, vitamin C and B vitamins as well as insoluble fibre.

CHAPTER 14

HEALTHY AGING

There might be a purpose for all species to not attain immortality. However that certainly does not mean that as we chronologically age, we should do so in pain and suffering. There are a lot of other animal species which mature and reach the end of their lives without being afflicted by biological disabilities faced by human beings. For example lobsters, rock-fish and tortoises among others, do not display signs of biological aging. Yes, we are not lobsters but there is absolutely no reason why we should also not age in a healthy way and be healthy until the end of our lifespan.

Healthy aging is classified as chronological aging which is accompanied by as little discomfort from age related conditions as possible. When people age in a healthy way, they have the opportunity to continue doing what they love and lead a high quality of life throughout their lives. An ideal person who ages in a healthy way is free from sicknesses and disorders for as long as possible and can continue being productive for much longer. A healthy aged adult is not a burden to society but is an active contributor to its advancement. They are mentally and physically active and competent for long.

A number of people have been able to attain healthy aging through following some basic recommendations. Studying these people shows that they follow certain lifestyles and good habits which keep them healthy for longer. Some habits of healthy agers are discussed briefly below.

Regular exercise

Most healthy agers lead an active life. Some follow systemic exercise routines while others lead active lives as a result of cultural activities or a different lifestyle. Exercise has a number of benefits which slow down the aging process. Some of these benefits include:

- Stronger muscles and bones.
- An increase in muscle mass.
- Adequate blood circulation.
- Improved waste removal.
- Well-functioning joints and ligaments.
- Lower risks of developing heart and circulation related problems.

- Reduces the risk of developing some age related diseases

- Boosts the immune system.

- Reduced stress and anxiety.

- Maintaining a healthy weight.

Falls are quite common with age. Exercises can help with balance and preventing injuries related to falls. Some chronic conditions like arthritis, high-blood pressure, diabetes and heart disease have been shown to improve with exercise. It is never too late to start exercising. However the earlier one starts the better.

Maintaining a healthy weight

A healthy weight has been shown to increase one's health. Keeping a healthy weight can greatly contribute to healthy aging. With a number of health conditions associated with obesity, watching one's weight might improve health and prevent some weight gain related conditions such as type 2 diabetes, stroke and high blood pressure. Watching weight includes being vigilant against being underweight as well. Underweight individuals tend to have a lower lifespan. Fat distribution must be closely monitored. Weight around the waist is dangerous and has been linked to increased risks of developing heart diseases.

The nutrition connection

Nutrition plays a huge role in healthy aging. The type of food one eats can affect not only health but fat distribution as well. As mentioned above, it is important to maintain a healthy weight and also maintain a healthy shape. Plant based foods are high in phytochemicals antioxidant and anti-inflammation compounds. Colourful fruits and vegetables are high in these amazing compounds as well as vitamins and minerals.

Healthy fats found in Avocados, nuts seeds, olives, olive oil and sardines are beneficial in healthy aging. Healthy fats are high in omega 3.Omega 3 fats are anti-inflammatory. Their counterparts, omega 6 fatty acids are pro inflammatory. A good balance between omega 3 and 6 will lead to a reduction in inflammation.

The importance of including fibre in the diet cannot be stressed enough. Soluble fibre is highly beneficial in cultivation and promoting the growth of healthy gut bacteria. A healthy gut has also been shown to support immune function. More benefits of healthy eating are outlined in the digestive health section.

In order to maintain healthy eating habits, it is important to:

- Manage caloric intake
- Avoid processed foods
- Adopt a plant based diet
- Eat high quality proteins
- Reduce processed carbohydrates
- Increase fibre rich foods
- Avoid sugar and sweetened beverages

The stress connection

Stress not only contributes to illnesses and disease. It can make one age much faster. People in stressful conditions tend to exhibit aging signs quicker than less stressed individuals. In order to maintain a stress free life, it is important to:

- Cultivate hobbies and do activities you enjoy.
- Stay connected and keep the mind busy and active.

- Spend time with people who make you happy.

- Avoid stressful environments and conditions.

- Practice taking good quality sleep.

Minimising age related illnesses

One of the biggest concerns with aging are all the age related diseases and disorders. Some healthy habits mentioned above are beneficial in eliminating and reducing age related disorders. Staying healthy can delay the onset of debilitating age related disorders. Indeed there are some conditions we do not have control over. However, preventing the ones we can will make a huge difference. Early detection and treatment of certain conditions may also reduce the chances of disability.

Aging solutions might not necessarily extend life but may increase the quality of life and delay the onset of debilitating age related conditions. Merely extending the life of a person by stretching chronological age without improving the quality of life and delaying the onset of age related disabilities prolong pain and suffering.

A good quality of life at old age benefits more people. The younger we stay the more we can contribute to society. As the quality of life increases, productive individuals remain beneficial to society for longer. Having healthier adults also reduces the burden on health systems and society.